Lean and Green Diet Cookbook

50 Quick and Easy Recipes to Enjoy. Lean and Green Diet Meals to Burn Fat and Stay Healthy Without Exercise. Regain Your Body Shape with the Fat-Burning Power of these Common Ingredients

By **Sophie Cook**

Table of Contents

Additionally, the information in the following pages is intended only for informational purposes and should thus be thought of as universal. As befitting its nature, it is presented without assurance regarding its prolonged validity or interim quality. Trademarks that are mentioned are done without written consent and can in no way be considered an endorsement from the trademark holder.

Introduction

The Lean and green diet is designed to help people lose weight and fat by reducing calories and carbohydrates through portion-controlled meals and snacks.

Between 6 portioned-controlled meals, the 5&1 plan limits the calories to 800-1,000 calories per day.

A lot of researches also revealed that reducing the total intake of calories is effective for weight loss. The low-carb diets are also included here.

A study was conducted for 16 weeks, having 198 participants with excess weight or obesity. They found out that Lean and Green 5&1 Plan had significantly lower weight, waist circumference, and fat levels than the control group.

The research suggested additional benefits since it resulted in the right way. It associates 5-10 % weight loss with a reduced risk of heart disease and also types two diabetes. Those who also tried the 5&1 Plan lost 5.7% of their body weight, on average, having a percentage of 28.1 % of participants losing over 105.

It is also said that one-on-one coaching is constructive, as well. A similar study was also conducted regarding it. They found out that individuals on the 5&1 diet who have completed at least 75% of the coaching sessions had lost more than twice their original weight, unlike those who only participated in fewer sessions.

All the same, many significant and related studies have also demonstrated and resulted in a substantial improvement with short and long-term weight loss. The diet adherence in programs that includes ongoing coaching is also included in it.

But then, currently, there are no studies yet that have proven the long-term results of the Lean and Green diet. Still, research conducted similar to a diet plan noted that the percentage of participants who have maintained the diet for a year was 25%.

Another research also showed some of them regain weight during the weight maintenance phase while following another diets. Coaching is the only factor that differs from these 5&1 diets and the 5&1 Lean and Green Plan. Overall, it is inevitable that more research is needed to assess the Lean and Green diet's lifetime effectiveness.

The low calorie and low carbohydrates plan of this diet is continuously gathering support from experts since it has been proven to show temporary fat and weight loss. In the future, if more research and study will be done, its long-term effectiveness will now be defined.

The Lean and Green diet is considered a high-protein diet, having a protein that counts up to 10–35% of a person's daily calories. Nevertheless, powdered, processed substances can result in some unpleasant consequences.

According to London, "The additives and protein isolate plus can give you some unnecessary GI side effects that can make an individual feel bloated, making it a lot better with a sugar-free Greek yogurt that contains protein in a smoothie." Also, according to London, "there is no regulation of dietary supplements like powders and shakes for safety by the FDA as there is for foods. Protein blends and powders can contain unwanted ingredients and can interfere with your medication. This makes it important to inform your doctor about what you are trying to indulge yourself in".

Chapter 1. What Is Lean and Green Diet

The Lean and Green Diet encourages people to limit the number of calories that they should take daily. Under this program, dieters are encouraged to consume between 800 and 1000 calories daily. For this to be possible, dieters are encouraged to opt for healthier food items and meal replacements. But unlike other types of commercial diet regimens, the Lean and Green Diet comes in different variations. There are currently three variations of this diet plan that one can choose according to one's needs.

- 5&1 Lean and Green Diet Plan: This is the most common version of this diet, and it involves eating five prepackaged meals from the Optimal Health Fueling and one home-made balanced dinner.

- 4&2&1 Lean and Green Diet Plan: This diet plan is designed for people who want to have flexibility while following this regimen. Under this program, dieters are encouraged to eat more calories and have more flexible food choices. This means that they can consume four prepackaged Optimal Health Fueling food, three home-cooked meals from the Lean and Green, and one snack daily.

- 5&2&2 Lean and Green Diet Plan: This diet plan is perfect for individuals who prefer to have a flexible meal plan to achieve a healthy weight. It is recommended for a wide variety of people. Under this diet regimen, dieters must eat five fueling, two lean and green meals, and two healthy snacks.

- 3&3 Lean and Green Diet Plan: This particular Diet plan is created for people who have moderate weight problems and merely want to maintain a healthy body. Under this diet plan, dieters are encouraged to consume three prepackaged Optimal Health Fuelings and three home-cooked meals.
- Lean and Green for Nursing Mothers: This diet regimen is designed for nursing mothers with babies of at least two months old. Aside from supporting breastfeeding mothers, it also encourages gradual weight loss.
- Lean and Green for Diabetes: This is designed for Type 1 and Type 2 diabetes people. The meal plans are designed to consume more green and lean meals, depending on their needs and condition.
- Lean and Green for Gout: This diet regimen incorporates a balance of low in purines and moderate in protein.
- Lean and Green for seniors (65 years and older): Designed for seniors, this diet plan has some variations following the components of Fuelings depending on the senior dieters' needs and activities.
- Lean and Green for Teen Boys and Teen Girls (13-18 years old): Designed for active teens, this diet for Teen Boys and Teen Girls provides the right nutrition to growing teens.

Regardless of which type of Lean and Green Diet plan you choose, you must talk with a coach to determine which program is right for you based on your individual goals. This is to ensure that you get the most out of the plan that you have chosen.

How to Start This Diet

The Lean and Green Diet is comprised of different phases. A certified coach will educate you on the steps you need to undertake to follow this regimen. But for the sake of those who are new to this diet, below are some of the things that you need to know, especially when you are still starting with this diet regimen.

Initial Steps

During this phase, people are encouraged to consume 800 to 1,000 calories to help them shed off at least 12 pounds within the next 12 weeks. For instance, if you are following the 5&1 Diet Plan, you need to eat a meal every 40 minutes and include a 30-minute moderate workout on most days of your week. You need to consume not more than 100 grams of Carbohydrates daily during this phase.

Further, consuming lean and green meals is highly encouraged. It involves eating 5 to 7 ounces of cooked lean proteins, three servings of non-starchy vegetables, and two healthy fats. This phase also encourages the dieter to include one optional snack per day, such as 1/2 cup sugar-free gelatin, three celery sticks, and 12 ounces nuts. Aside from these things, below are other things that you need to remember when following this phase:

- Make sure that the portion size recommendations are for cooked weight and not the raw -weight of your ingredients
- Opt for meals that are baked, grilled, broiled, or poached. Avoid frying foods, as this will increase your calorie intake.

- Eat at least two servings of fish rich in Omega-3 fatty acids. These include fishes like tuna, salmon, trout, mackerel, herring, and other cold-water fishes.
-Choose meatless alternatives like tofu and tempeh.
-Follow the program even when you are dining out. Keep in mind that drinking alcohol is discouraged when following this plan.

Maintenance Phase

As soon as you have achieved your desired weight, the next phase is the transition stage. It is a 6-week stage that involves increasing your calorie intake to 1,550 per day. This is also the phase when you can add more varieties into your meal, such as whole grains, low-fat dairy, and fruits.
After six weeks, you can now move into the 3&3 Lean and Green Diet plan, so you are required to eat three lean and green meals and 3 Fueling foods.

Chapter 2. How It Works

The Lean and Green Diet is viewed as a high-protein diet, with its protein having 10–35% of your daily calories. Be that as it may, the handled, powdered kind can prompt some not exactly beautiful outcomes. "The protein confine in addition to added substances can cause you to feel enlarged and have caused some undesirable GI symptoms, making you off with unsweetened Greek yogurt for protein in a single smoothie," London says.

The FDA also doesn't direct dietary enhancements like shakes and powders for security and viability in a similar way it accomplishes for food. "Powders and protein 'mixes' may have unwanted fixings, or could interface with a drug you might be taking," London includes, "making it extra critical to ensure your doctor knows about you attempting the arrangement."

Like many commercial plans, this one involves buying most of the foods permitted on a diet in packaged form. The company deals in a wide range of food products that they call "fuelings"—on its website. These include pancakes, shakes, pasta dishes, soups, cookies, mashed potatoes, and popcorn.

Users pick the plan that best suits them. The 5 & 1 Plan entails eating five small meals per day. The meals can be selected from more than 60 substitutable fuelings, including one lean and green meal, probably veggies or protein that you will prepare by yourself. The Optimal Essential Kit, costing $356.15, provides 119 servings, or about 20 days' worth.

A flexible option is the 4 & 2 & 1 Plan. It merely contains four daily fuelings; you can choose and create two of your own lean and green meals and one of the purchased snacks. Also, including a similar mix of convenience food, a kit with 140 servings costs $399.00.

How Much Does Lean and Green Cost?

In comparison, the United States Department of Agriculture estimates that a woman whose ages range from 10-50 can follow a nutritious diet while spending as little as $166.40 per month on groceries. As long as she is preparing all her meals at home.

How Nutritious Is This Diet

Below is the breakdown comparison of meals' nutritional content on the Lean and Green Weight 5&1 Plan and the federal government's 2015 Dietary Guidelines for Americans.

	Optimal Weight 5&1 Plan	**Federal Government Recommendation**
Calories	800-1,000	Men 19-25: 2,800 26-45: 2,600 46-65: 2,400 65+: 2,200 Women 19-25: 2,200 26-50: 2,000 51+: 1,800
Total fat **% of Calorie Intake**	20%	20%-35%

Total Carbohydrates **% of Calorie Intake**	40%	45%-65%
Sugars	10%-20%	N/A
Fiber	25 g – 30 g	Men 19-30: 34 g. 31-50: 31 g. 51+: 28 g. Women 19-30: 28 g. 31-50: 25 g. 51+: 22 g.
Protein	40%	10%-35%
Sodium	Under 2,300 mg	Under 2,300 mg.
Potassium	Average 3,000 mg	At least 4,700 mg.
Calcium	1,000 mg – 1,200 mg	Men 1,000 mg. Women 19-50: 1,000 mg. 51+: 1,200 mg.

Chapter 3. Breakfast

Millet Porridge

Preparation Time: 10 minutes
Cooking Time: 20 minutes
Servings: 2
Ingredients:

- Sea salt
- 1 tbsp. finely chopped coconuts
- 1/2 cup unsweetened coconut milk
- 1/2 cup rinsed and drained millet
- 1-1/2 cups alkaline water
- 3 drops liquid stevia

Directions:

1. Sauté the millet in a non-stick skillet for about 3 minutes.
2. Add salt and water then stir.
3. Let the meal boil then reduce the amount of heat.
4. Cook for 15 minutes then add the remaining ingredients. Stir.
5. Cook the meal for 4 extra minutes.
6. Serve the meal with toping of the chopped nuts.

Nutrition:
Calories: 219 kcal
Fat: 4.5g
Carbs: 38.2g
Protein: 6.4g

Jackfruit Vegetable Fry

Preparation Time: 5 minutes
Cooking Time: 5 minutes
Servings: 6
Ingredients:

- 2 finely chopped small onions
- 2 cups finely chopped cherry tomatoes
- 1/8 tsp. ground turmeric
- 1 tbsp. olive oil
- 2 seeded and chopped red bell peppers
- 3 cups seeded and chopped firm jackfruit
- 1/8 tsp. cayenne pepper
- 2 tbsps. chopped fresh basil leaves
- Salt

Directions:

1. In a greased skillet, sauté the onions and bell peppers for about 5 minutes.
2. Add the tomatoes then stir.
3. Cook for 2 minutes.
4. Then add the jackfruit, cayenne pepper, salt, and turmeric.
5. Cook for about 8 minutes.
6. Garnish the meal with basil leaves.
7. Serve warm.

Nutrition:
Calories: 236 kcal
Fat: 1.8g
Carbs: 48.3g
Protein: 7g

Chapter 4. Lunch

Bacon and Egg Quesadillas

Preparation Time: 10 minutes
Cooking time: 30 minutes
Servings: 3
Ingredients:

- 8 low carb tortilla shells
- 6 eggs
- 1 cup water
- 3 tablespoon butter
- 1 ½ cups grated cheddar cheese
- 1 ½ cups grated Swiss cheese
- 5 bacon slices
- 1 medium onion, thinly sliced
- 1 tablespoon chopped parsley

Directions

1. Bring the eggs to a boil in water over medium heat for 10 minutes. Transfer the eggs to an ice water bath, peel the shells, and chop them; set aside.
2. Meanwhile, as the eggs cook, fry the bacon in a skillet over medium heat for 4 minutes until crispy. Remove and chop. Plate and set aside too.
3. Fetch out 2/3 of the bacon fat and sauté the onions in the remaining grease over medium heat for 2 minutes; set aside. Melt 1 tablespoon of butter in a skillet over medium heat.
4. Lay one tortilla in a skillet; sprinkle with some Swiss cheese. Add some chopped eggs and bacon over the cheese, top with onion, and sprinkle with some cheddar

cheese. Cover with another tortilla shell. Cook for 45 seconds, then carefully flip the quesadilla, and cook the other side too for 45 seconds. Remove to a plate and repeat the cooking process using the remaining tortilla shells.

5. Garnish with parsley and serve warm.

Nutrition:
Kcal 449,
Fat 48.7g,
Net Carbs 6.8g,
Protein 29.1g

Avocado and Kale Eggs

Preparation Time: 10 minutes
Cooking time: 30 minutes
Servings: 3
Ingredients:

- 1 teaspoon ghee
- 1 red onion, sliced
- 4 oz chorizo, sliced into thin rounds
- 1 cup chopped kale
- 1 ripe avocado, pitted, peeled, chopped
- 4 eggs
- Salt and black pepper to season

Directions:

1. Preheat oven to 370°F.
2. Melt ghee in a cast iron pan over medium heat and sauté the onion for 2 minutes. Add the chorizo and cook for 2 minutes more, flipping once.
3. Introduce the kale in batches with a splash of water to wilt, season lightly with salt, stir and cook for 3 minutes. Mix in the avocado and turn the heat off.
4. Create four holes in the mixture, crack the eggs into each hole, sprinkle with salt and black pepper, and slide the pan into the preheated oven to bake for 6 minutes until the egg whites are set or firm and yolks still runny. Season to taste with salt and pepper, and serve right away with low carb toasts.

Nutrition:

Kcal 274,
Fat 23g,
Net Carbs 4g,
Protein 13g

Bacon and Cheese Frittata

Preparation Time: 10 minutes
Cooking time: 20 minutes
Servings: 3
Ingredients:

- 10 slices bacon
- 10 fresh eggs
- 3 tablespoon butter, melted
- ½ cup almond milk
- Salt and black pepper to taste
- 1 ½ cups cheddar cheese, shredded
- ¼ cup chopped green onions

Directions:

1. Preheat the oven to 400°F and grease a baking dish with cooking spray. Cook the bacon in a skillet over medium heat for 6 minutes. Once crispy, remove from the skillet to paper towels and discard grease. Chop into small pieces. Whisk the eggs, butter, milk, salt, and black pepper. Mix in the bacon and pour the mixture into the baking dish.

2. Sprinkle with cheddar cheese and green onions, and bake in the oven for 10 minutes or until the eggs are thoroughly cooked. Remove and cool the frittata for 3 minutes, slice into wedges, and serve warm with a dollop of Greek yogurt.

Nutrition:

Kcal 325,
Fat 28g,
Net Carbs 2g,
Protein 15g

Spicy Egg Muffins with Bacon & Cheese

Preparation Time: 10 minutes
Cooking time: 20 minutes
Servings: 3
Ingredients:

- 12 eggs
- ¼ cup coconut milk
- Salt and black pepper to taste
- 1 cup grated cheddar cheese
- 12 slices bacon
- 4 jalapeño peppers, seeded and minced

Directions:

1. Preheat oven to 370°F.
2. Crack the eggs into a bowl and whisk with coconut milk until combined. Season with salt and pepper, and evenly stir in the cheddar cheese.
3. Line each hole of a muffin tin with a slice of bacon and fill each with the egg mixture two-thirds way up. Top with the jalapeno peppers and bake in the oven for 18 to 20 minutes or until puffed and golden. Remove, allow cooling for a few minutes, and serve with arugula salad.

Nutrition:
Kcal 302,
Fat 23.7g,
Net Carbs 3.2g,
Protein 20g

Chapter 5. Dinner

Bacon & Chicken Patties

Preparation Time: 5 minutes
Cooking Time: 15 minutes
Servings: 2
Ingredients:

- 1 ½ oz. can chicken breast
- 4 slices bacon
- ¼ cup parmesan cheese
- 1 large egg
- 3 tbsp. flour

Directions:

1. Cook the bacon until crispy.
2. Chop the chicken and bacon together in a food processor until fine.
3. Add in the parmesan, egg, flour and mix.
4. Make the patties by hand and fry on a medium heat in a pan with some oil.
5. Once browned, flip over, continue cooking, and lie them to drain.
6. Serve!

Nutrition:
Calories: 387
Carbs: 13 g
Fat: 16 g
Protein: 34 g
Fiber: 28 g

Cheddar Bacon Burst

Preparation Time: 25 minutes
Cooking Time: 40 minutes
Servings: 8
Ingredients:

- 30 slices bacon
- 2 ½ cups cheddar cheese
- 4-5 cups raw spinach
- 1-2 tbsp. Tones Southwest Chipotle Seasoning
- 2 tsp Mrs. Dash Table Seasoning

Directions:

1. Preheat your fryer to 375°F/190°C.
2. Weave the bacon into 15 vertical pieces & 12 horizontal pieces. Cut the extra 3 in half to fill in the rest, horizontally.
3. Season the bacon.
4. Add the cheese to the bacon.
5. Add the spinach and press down to compress.
6. Tightly roll up the woven bacon.
7. Line a baking sheet with kitchen foil and add plenty of salt to it.
8. Put the bacon on top of a cooling rack and put that on top of your baking sheet.
9. Bake for 30-40 minutes.
10. Let cool for 10-15 minutes before
11. Slice and enjoy!

Nutrition:
Calories: 218
Carbs: 20 g
Fat: 9 g
Protein: 21 g
Fiber: 5 g

Grilled Ham & Cheese

Preparation Time: 15 minutes
Cooking Time: 30 minutes
Servings: 2
Ingredients:

- 3 low-carb buns
- 4 slices medium-cut deli ham
- 1 tbsp. salted butter
- 1 oz. flour
- 3 slices cheddar cheese
- 3 slices muenster cheese

Directions:
Bread:

1. Preheat your fryer to 350°F/175°C.
2. Mix the flour, salt and baking powder in a bowl. Put to the side.
3. Add in the butter and coconut oil to a skillet.
4. Melt for 20 seconds and pour into another bowl.
5. In this bowl, mix in the dough.
6. Scramble two eggs. Add to the dough.
7. Add ½ tablespoon of coconut flour to thicken, and place evenly into a cupcake tray. Fill about ¾ inch.
8. Bake for 20 minutes until browned.
9. Allow to cool for 15 minutes and cut each in half for the buns.

Sandwich:

1. Fry the deli meat in a skillet on a high heat.
2. Put the ham and cheese between the buns.
3. Heat the butter on medium high.
4. When brown, turn to low and add the dough to pan.
5. Press down with a weight until you smell burning, then flip to crisp both sides.
6. Enjoy!

Nutrition:
Calories: 188
Carbs: 12 g
Fat: 16 g
Protein: 14 g
Fiber: 18 g

Prosciutto Spinach Salad

Preparation Time: 5 minutes
Cooking Time: 5 minutes
Servings: 2
Ingredients:

- 2 cups baby spinach
- 1/3 lb. prosciutto
- 1 cantaloupe
- 1 avocado
- ¼ cup diced red onion handful of raw, unsalted walnuts

Directions:

1. Put a cup of spinach on each plate.
2. Top with the diced prosciutto, cubes of balls of melon, slices of avocado, a handful of red onion and a few walnuts.
3. Add some freshly ground pepper, if you like.
4. Serve!

Nutrition:
Calories: 348
Carbs: 11 g
Fat: 9 g
Protein: 26 g
Fiber: 22 g

Chapter 6. Vegetable

Cauliflower and Egg Plate

Preparation Time: 5 minutes
Cooking Time: 12 minutes;
Servings: 2
Ingredients

- 4 oz cauliflower florets, chopped
- 1 jalapeno pepper, sliced
- 2 eggs
- 1 ½ tbsp. avocado oil
- Seasoning:
- ¼ tsp salt
- 1/8 tsp ground black pepper

Directions:

1. Take a skillet pan, place it over medium heat, add oil and when hot, add cauliflower florets and jalapeno and then cook for 5 to 7 minutes until tender.
2. Make two spaces in the pan, crack an egg in each space, and then cook for 3 to 4 minutes until eggs have cooked to the desired level.
3. When done, sprinkle salt and black pepper over eggs and then serve.

Nutrition:
191 Calories;
16 g Fats;
11 g Protein;
2 g Net Carb;
0 g Fiber

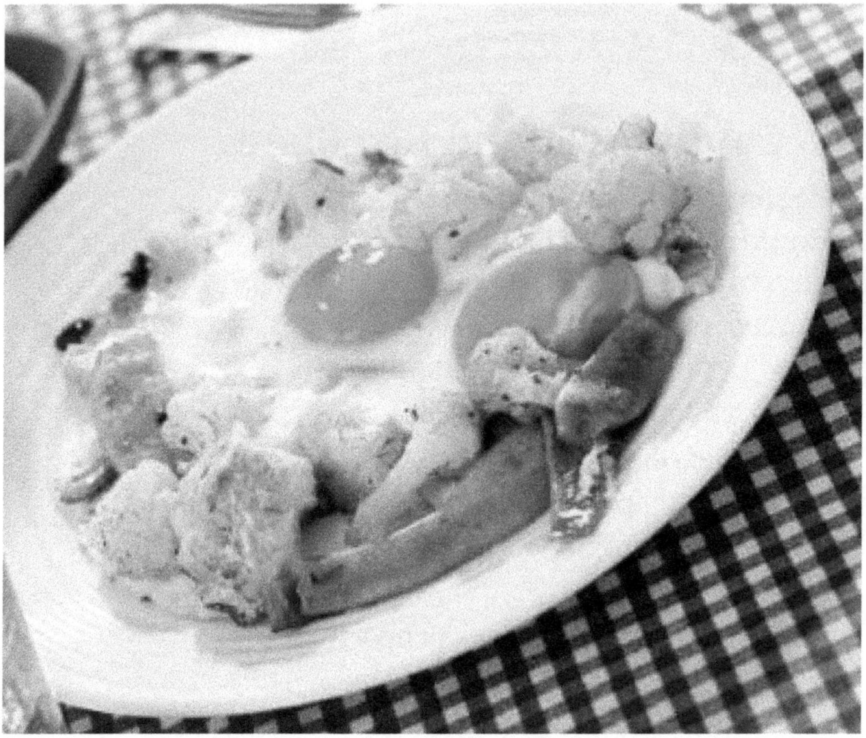

Butternut Squash and Green Onions with Eggs

Preparation Time: 5 minutes
Cooking Time: 8 minutes;
Servings: 2
Ingredients

- 4 oz butternut squash pieces
- 1 green onion, sliced
- ½ tbsp. butter, unsalted
- 2 tsp grated parmesan cheese
- 2 eggs
- Seasoning:
- ¼ tsp salt
- ¼ tsp ground black pepper
- 1 tsp avocado oil

Directions:

1. Take a skillet pan, place it over medium heat, add butter and oil and when hot, add butternut squash and green onion, season with 1/8 tsp of each salt and black pepper, stir until mixed and cook for 3 to 5 minutes until tender.

2. Make two space in the pan, crack an egg in each space, and sprinkle with cheese, season with remaining salt and black pepper, cover with the lid and cook for 2 to 3 minutes until the egg has cooked to the desired level.

3. Serve.

Nutrition:
191 Calories;
16 g Fats;
11 g Protein;
2 g Net Carb;
0 g Fiber

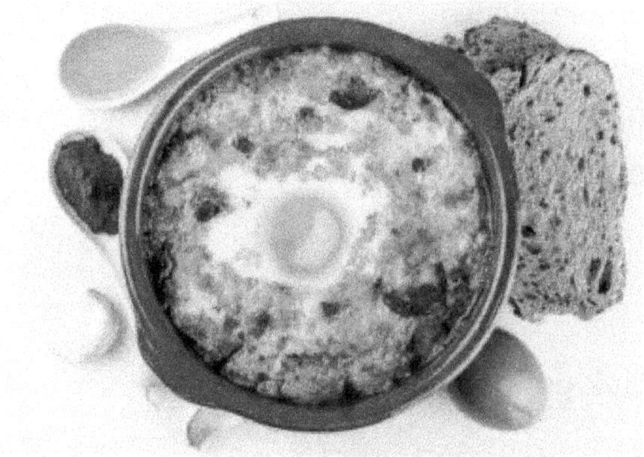

Broccoli, Asparagus and Cheese Frittata

Preparation Time: 5 minutes
Cooking Time: 16 minutes;
Servings: 2
Ingredients

- ¼ cup chopped broccoli florets
- 1-ounce asparagus spear cuts
- ½ tsp garlic powder
- 2 tbsp. whipping cream
- 2 eggs
- Seasoning:
- 2 tsp tbsp. avocado oil
- 1/8 tsp salt
- 1/8 tsp ground black pepper

Directions:

1. Turn on the oven, then set it to 350 degrees F and let it preheat.
2. Take a medium bowl, crack eggs in it, add salt, black pepper and cream, whisk until combined and then stir in cheese, set aside until required.
3. Take a medium skillet pan, place it over medium heat, add oil and when hot, add broccoli florets and asparagus, sprinkle with garlic powder, stir until mixed and cook for 3 to 4 minutes until tender.
4. Spread the vegetables evenly in the pan, pour egg mixture over them and cook for 1 to 2 minutes until the mixture begins to firm.

5. Transfer the pan into the oven and then cook for 10 to 12 minutes until frittata has cooked and the top has turned golden brown.
6. When done, cut the frittata into slices and then serve.

Nutrition:
206 Calories;
17 g Fats;
10 g Protein;
2 g Net Carb;
1 g Fiber;

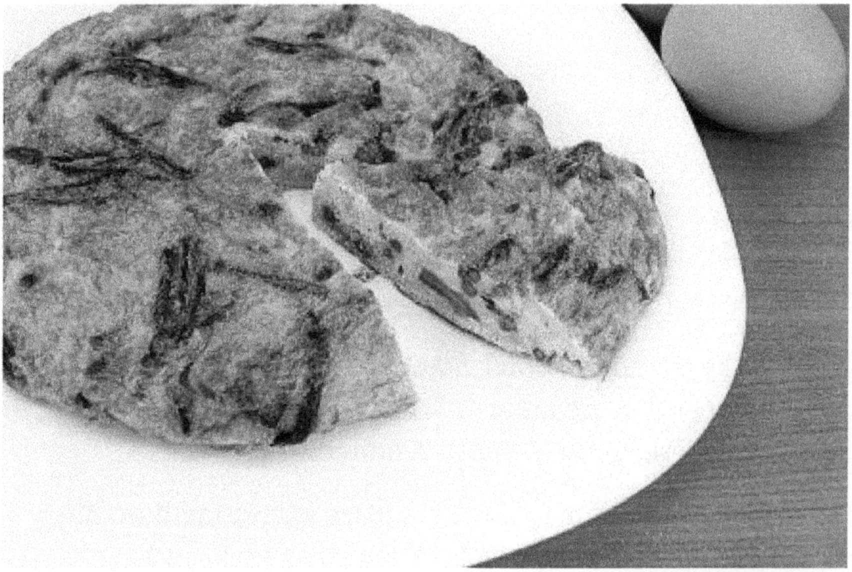

Broccoli and Egg Plate

Preparation Time: 5 minutes
Cooking Time: 5 minutes;
Servings: 2
Ingredients

- 3 oz broccoli florets, chopped
- 2 eggs
- 1 tbsp. avocado oil
- ¼ tsp salt
- 1/8 tsp ground black pepper

Directions:

1. Take a heatproof bowl, place broccoli florets in it, cover with a plastic wrap, microwave for 2 minutes, and then drain well.
2. Take a medium skillet pan, place it over medium heat, add oil and when hot, add broccoli florets and cook for 2 minutes until golden brown.
3. Spread broccoli florets evenly in the pan crack eggs in the pan, sprinkle with salt and black pepper, cover with the lid and cook for 2 to 3 minutes until eggs have cooked to the desired level.
4. Serve.

Nutrition:
155 Calories;
12 g Fats;
8 g Protein;
1.6 g Net Carb;
1 g Fiber;

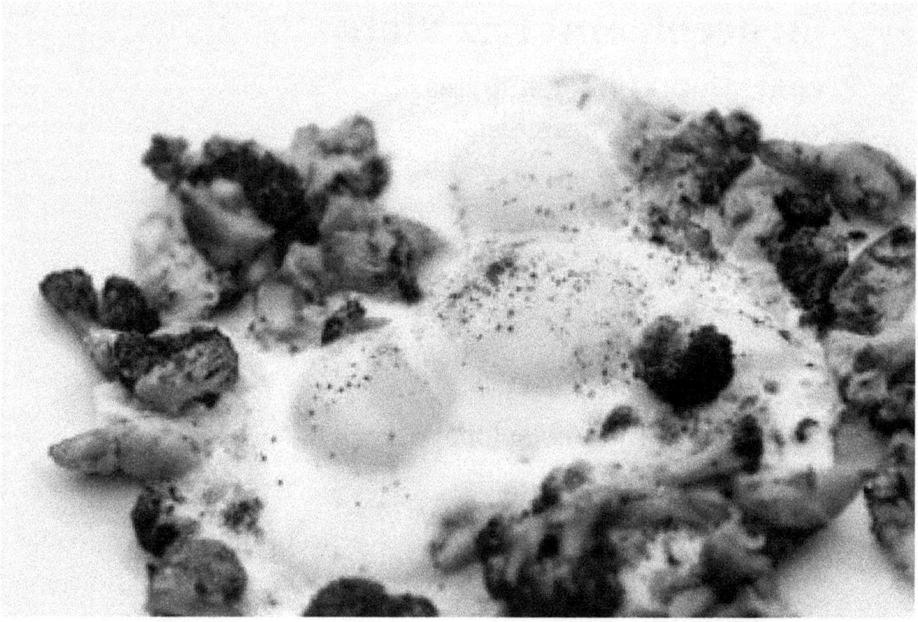

Radish with Fried Eggs

Preparation Time: 5 minutes
Cooking Time: 10 minutes;
Servings: 2
Ingredients

- ½ bunch of radish, diced
- ½ tsp garlic powder
- 1 tbsp. butter
- 1 tbsp. avocado oil
- 2 eggs
- Seasoning:
- 1/3 tsp salt
- ¼ tsp ground black pepper

Directions:

1. Take a medium skillet pan, place it over medium heat, add butter and when it melts, add radish, sprinkle with garlic powder and ¼ tsp salt and cook for 5 minutes until tender.
2. Distribute radish between two plates, then return pan over medium heat, add oil and when hot, crack eggs in it and fry for 2 to 3 minutes until cooked to desired level.
3. Add eggs to the radish and then serve.

Nutrition:
187 Calories;
17 g Fats;
7 g Protein;
0.4 g Net Carb;
0.5 g Fiber;

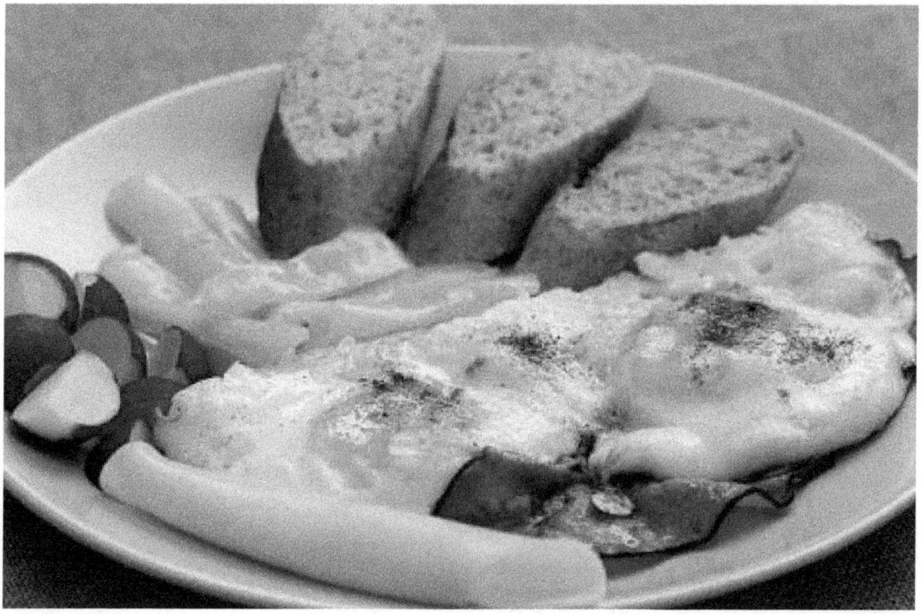

Sunny Side Up Eggs on Creamed Spinach

Preparation Time: 5 minutes
Cooking Time: 10 minutes;
Servings: 2
Ingredients

- 4 oz of spinach leaves
- 1 tbsp. mustard paste
- 4 tbsp. whipping cream
- 2 eggs
- Seasoning:
- ¼ tsp salt
- ¼ tsp ground black pepper
- ½ tsp dried thyme
- 1 tbsp. avocado oil

Directions:

1. Take a medium skillet pan, place it over high heat, pour in water to cover its bottom, then add spinach, toss until mixed and cook for 2 minutes until spinach wilts.
2. Then drain the spinach by passing it through a sieve placed on a bowl and set it aside.
3. Take a medium saucepan, place it over medium heat, add spinach, mustard, thyme, and cream, stir until mixed and cook for 2 minutes.
4. Then sprinkle black pepper over spinach, stir until mixed and remove the pan from heat.
5. Take a medium skillet pan, place it over medium-high heat, add oil and when hot, crack eggs in it and fry for 3 to 4 minutes until eggs have cooked to the desired level.

6. Divide spinach mixture evenly between two plates, top with a fried egg and then serve.

Nutrition:
280 Calories;
23.3 g Fats;
10.2 g Protein;
2.7 g Net Carb;
2.8 g Fiber;

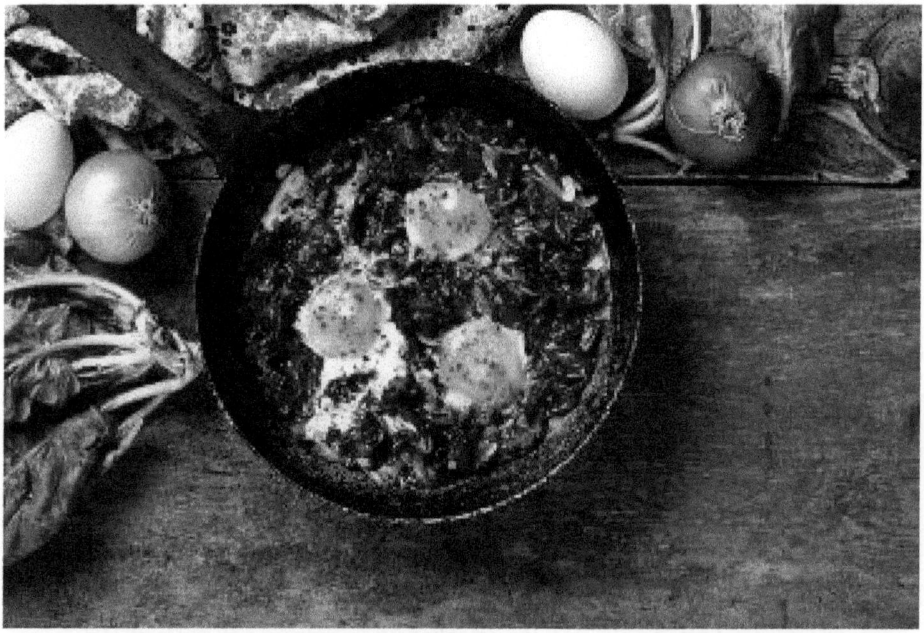

Chapter 7. Seafood

Saltine Fish Fillets

Preparation Time: 10 minutes
Cooking Time: 15 minutes
Servings: 4
Ingredients:

- 1 cup crushed saltines
- 1/4 cup extra-virgin olive oil
- 1 tsp. garlic powder
- 1/2 tsp. shallot powder
- 1 egg, well whisked
- 4 white fish fillets
- Salt and ground black pepper to taste
- Fresh Italian parsley to serve

Directions:

1. In a shallow bowl, combine the crushed saltines and olive oil.
2. In a separate bowl, mix together the garlic powder, shallot powder, and the beaten egg.
3. Sprinkle a good amount of salt and pepper over the fish, before dipping each fillet into the egg mixture.
4. Coat the fillets with the crumb mixture.
5. Air fry the fish at 370°F for 10 - 12 minutes.
6. Serve with fresh parsley.

Nutrition:
Calories: 502
Fat: 4g
Protein: 11g
Sugar: 9g

Air Fried Cod with Basil Vinaigrette

Preparation Time: 5 minutes
Cooking Time: 15 minutes
Servings: 4
Ingredients:

- ¼ cup olive oil
- 4 cod fillets
- A bunch of basil, torn
- Juice from 1 lemon, freshly squeezed
- Salt and pepper to taste

Directions:

1. Preheat the air fryer for 5 minutes.
2. Season the cod fillets with salt and pepper to taste.
3. Place in the air fryer and cook for 15 minutes at 350oF.
4. Meanwhile, mix the rest of the ingredients in a bowl and toss to combine.
5. Serve the air fried cod with the basil vinaigrette.

Nutrition:
Calories 235
Carbohydrates: 1.9g
Protein: 14.3g
Fat: 18.9g

Almond Flour Coated Crispy Shrimps

Preparation Time: 5 minutes
Cooking Time: 10 minutes
Servings: 4
Ingredients:

- ½ cup almond flour
- 1 tablespoon yellow mustard
- 1-pound raw shrimps, peeled and deveined
- 3 tablespoons olive oil
- Salt and pepper to taste

Directions:

1. Place all ingredients in a Ziploc bag and give a good shake.
2. Place in the air fryer and cook for 10 minutes at 4000F.

Nutrition:
Calories 206
Carbohydrates: 1.3g
Protein: 23.5g
Fat: 11.9g

Another Crispy Coconut Shrimp Recipe

Preparation Time: 5 minutes
Cooking Time: 20 minutes
Servings: 4
Ingredients:

- ½ cup flour
- ½ stick cold butter, cut into cubes
- ½ tablespoon lemon juice
- 1 egg yolk, beaten
- 1 green onion, chopped
- 1-pound salmon fillets, cut into small cubes
- 3 tablespoons whipping cream
- 4 eggs, beaten
- Salt and pepper to taste

Directions:

1. Preheat the air fryer to 3900F.
2. Season salmon fillets with lemon juice, salt and pepper.
3. In another bowl, combine the flour and butter. Add cold water gradually to form a dough. Knead the dough on a flat surface to form a sheet.
4. Place the dough on the baking dish and press firmly on the dish.
5. Beat the eggs and egg yolk and season with salt and pepper to taste.
6. Place the salmon cubes on the pan lined with dough and pour the egg over.
7. Cook for 15 to 20 minutes.

8. Garnish with green onions once cooked.

Nutrition:
Calories 483
Carbs: 5.2g
Protein: 45.2g
Fat: 31.2g

Chapter 8. Soup and Stew

"Ramen" Soup

Preparation Time: 10 minutes
Cooking Time: 15 minutes
Servings: 2 servings
Ingredients:

- 1 zucchini, trimmed
- 2 cups chicken broth
- 2 eggs, boiled, peeled
- 1 tablespoon coconut amines
- 5 oz. beef loin, strips
- 1 teaspoon chili flakes
- 1 tablespoon chives, chopped
- ½ teaspoon salt

Directions:

1. Put the beef loin strips in the instant pot.
2. Add chili flakes, salt, and chicken broth.
3. Close and seal the lid. Cook the Ingredients: on manual mode (high pressure) for 15 minutes. Make a quick pressure release and open the lid.
4. Then make the s from zucchini with the help of the spiralizer and add them in the soup.
5. Add chives and coconut aminos.
6. Then ladle the soup in the bowls and top with halved eggs.

Nutrition:
Calories 254
Fat 11.8
Fiber 1.1
Carbs 6.2
Protein 30.6

Beef Tagine

Preparation Time: 15 minutes
Cooking Time: 25 minutes
Servings: 6 servings
Ingredients:

- 1-pound beef fillet, chopped
- 1 eggplant, chopped
- 6 oz. scallions, chopped
- 1 teaspoon ground allspices
- 1 teaspoon Erythritol
- 1 teaspoon coconut oil
- 4 cups beef broth

Directions:

1. Put all Ingredients in the instant pot.
2. Close and seal the lid.
3. Cook the meal on manual mode (high pressure) for 25 minutes.
4. Then allow the natural pressure release for 15 minutes.

Nutrition:
Calories 146
Fat 5.3
Fiber 3.5
Carbs 8.8
Protein 16.7

Tomatillos Fish Stew

Preparation Time: 15 minutes
Cooking Time: 12 minutes
Servings: 2 servings
Ingredients:

- 2 tomatillos, chopped
- 10 oz. salmon fillet, chopped
- 1 teaspoon ground paprika
- ½ teaspoon ground turmeric
- 1 cup coconut cream
- ½ teaspoon salt

Directions:

1. Put all Ingredients in the instant pot.
2. Close and seal the lid.
3. Cook the fish stew on manual mode (high pressure) for 12 minutes.
4. Then allow the natural pressure release for 10 minutes.

Nutrition:
Calories 479
Fat 37.9
Fiber 3.8
Carbs 9.6
Protein 30.8

Chili Verde Soup

Preparation Time: 10 minutes
Cooking Time: 25 minutes
Servings: 4 servings
Ingredients:

- 2 oz. chili Verde sauce
- ½ cup Cheddar cheese, shredded
- 5 cups chicken broth
- 1-pound chicken breast, skinless, boneless
- 1 tablespoon dried cilantro

Directions:

1. Put chicken breast and chicken broth in the instant pot.
2. Add cilantro, close and seal the lid.
3. Then cook the Ingredients on manual (high pressure) for 15 minutes.
4. Make a quick pressure release and open the li.
5. Shred the chicken breast with the help of the fork.
6. Add dried cilantro and chili Verde sauce in the soup and cook it on saute mode for 10 minutes.
7. Then add dried cilantro and stir well.

Nutrition:
Calories 257
Fat 10.2
Fiber 0.2
Carbs 4
Protein 34.5

Chapter 9. Sides

Salmon Spinach and Cottage Cheese Sandwich

Preparation Time: 15 minutes
Cooking Time: 10 minutes
Servings: 4
Ingredients:

- 4 ounces (125 g) cottage cheese
- 1/4 cup (15 g) chives, chopped
- 1 teaspoon (5 g) capers
- 1/2 teaspoon (2.5 g) grated lemon rind
- 4 (2 oz. or 60 g) smoked salmon
- 2 cups (60 g) loose baby spinach
- 1 medium (110 g) red onion, sliced thinly
- 8 slices rye bread (about 30 g each)
- Kosher salt and freshly ground black pepper

Directions:

1. Preheat your griddle or Panini press.
2. Mix together cottage cheese, chives, capers, and lemon rind in a small bowl.
3. Spread and divide the cheese mixture on 4 bread slices. Top with spinach, onion slices, and smoked salmon.
4. Cover with remaining bread slices.
5. Grill the sandwiches until golden and grill marks form on both sides.
6. Transfer to a serving dish.
7. Serve and enjoy.

Nutrition:
Calories: 261
Fat 9.9 g
Carbohydrates 22.9 g
Protein 19.9 g
Sodium - 1226 mg

Salmon Feta and Pesto Wrap

Preparation Time: 15 minutes
Cooking Time: 10 minutes
Servings: 4
Ingredients:

- 8 ounces (250 g) smoked salmon fillet, thinly sliced
- 1 cup (150 g) feta cheese
- 8 (15 g) Romaine lettuce leaves
- 4 (6-inch) pita bread
- 1/4 cup (60 g) basil pesto sauce

Directions:

1. Place 1 pita bread on a plate. Top with lettuce, salmon, feta cheese, and pesto sauce. Fold or roll to enclose filling. Repeat procedure for the remaining ingredients.
2. Serve and enjoy.

Nutrition:
Calories: 379
Fat 17.7 g
Carbohydrates: 36.6 g
Protein: 18.4 g
Sodium: 554 mg

Salmon Cream Cheese and Onion on Bagel

Preparation Time: 15 minutes
Cooking Time: 10 minutes
Servings: 4
Ingredients:

- 8 ounces (250 g) smoked salmon fillet, thinly sliced
- 1/2 cup (125 g) cream cheese
- 1 medium (110 g) onion, thinly sliced
- 4 bagels (about 80g each), split
- 2 tablespoons (7 g) fresh parsley, chopped
- Freshly ground black pepper, to taste

Directions:

1. Spread the cream cheese on each bottom's half of bagels. Top with salmon and onion, season with pepper, sprinkle with parsley and then cover with bagel tops.
2. Serve and enjoy.

Nutrition:
Calories: 309
Fat 14.1 g
Carbohydrates 32.0 g
Protein 14.7 g
Sodium 571 mg

Chapter 10. Desserts

Minty Coconut Cream

Preparation Time: 4 minutes
Cooking Time: 0 minutes
Servings: 2
Ingredients:

- 1 banana, peeled
- 2 cups coconut flesh, shredded
- 3 tablespoons mint, chopped
- 1 and ½ cups coconut water
- 2 tablespoons stevia
- ½ avocado, pitted and peeled

Directions:

1. In a blender, combine the coconut with the banana and the rest of the ingredients, pulse well, divide into cups and serve cold.

Nutrition:
Calories 193
Fat 5.4
Fiber 3.4
Carbs 7.6
Protein 3

Grapes Stew

Preparation Time: 10 minutes
Cooking Time: 10 minutes
Servings: 4
Ingredients:

- 2/3 cup stevia
- 1 tablespoon olive oil
- 1/3 cup coconut water
- 1 teaspoon vanilla extract
- 1 teaspoon lemon zest, grated
- 2 cup red grapes, halved

Directions:

1. Heat up a pan with the water over medium heat, add the oil, stevia and the rest of the ingredients, toss, simmer for 10 minutes, divide into cups and serve.

Nutrition:
Calories 122
Fat 3.7
Fiber 1.2
Carbs 2.3
Protein 0.4

Cocoa Sweet Cherry Cream

Preparation Time: 40 minutes
Cooking Time: 0 minutes
Servings: 4
Ingredients:

- ½ cup cocoa powder
- ¾ cup red cherry jam
- ¼ cup stevia
- 2 cups water
- 1-pound cherries, pitted and halved

Directions:

1. In a blender, mix the cherries with the water and the rest of the ingredients, pulse well, divide into cups and keep in the fridge for 40 minutes before serving.

Nutrition:
Calories 162
Fat 3.4
Fiber 2.4
Carbs 5
Protein 1

Apple Couscous Pudding

Preparation Time: 10 minutes
Cooking Time: 25 minutes
Servings: 4
Ingredients:

- ½ cup couscous
- 1 and ½ cups milk
- ¼ cup apple, cored and chopped
- 3 tablespoons stevia
- ½ teaspoon rose water
- 1 tablespoon orange zest, grated

Directions:

1. Heat up a pan with the milk over medium heat,
2. add the couscous and the rest of the ingredients, whisk, simmer for 25 minutes, divide into bowls and serve.

Nutrition:

Calories 150
Fat 4.5
Fiber 5.5
Carbs 7.5
Protein 4

Chapter 11. Meat

Lamb Meatballs with Feta

Preparation Time: 5 minutes
Cooking Time: 30 minutes
Servings: 4
Ingredients:

- 0,33 lb lamb minces
- 1 slice of stale white bread, turned into fine crumbs
- 0,11 lb Greek feta, crumbled
- 1 tablespoon fresh oregano, finely chopped
- ½ tablespoon grated lemon peel
- Freshly ground black pepper

Directions:

1. Preheat the Air Fryer to 392 ° F.
2. Mix the mince in a bowl with the bread crumbs, feta, oregano, lemon peel and black pepper, thoroughly kneading everything together.
3. Cut the mixture in 10 equal portions to make round balls.
4. Place this dish in the basket after putting them in the oven dish. Slide the basket into the Air Fryer. Set the timer to 8 minutes and bake the mince balls until they are nicely brown and done.
5. Serve the meatballs hot in a platter with tapas forks

Nutrition:
Calories: 300
Fat: 2.5g
Carbs: 5g
Protein: 13g

Garlic Lamb with Rosemary

Preparation Time: 5 minutes
Cooking Time: 40 minutes
Servings: 4
Ingredients:

- 1 leg of lamb
- Branches of fresh rosemary
- Several garlic cloves
- 5 pepper (or otherwise black pepper)
- Fleur de sel
- 2 onions
- 2,2 lb of potatoes
- Extra virgin olive oil

Directions:

1. Preheat the Air fryer to 356 ° F.
2. Remove the blade bone of the lamb. Remove excess fat.
3. Dry the piece of blood residues. If you removed the bone, salt and pepper inside and close to giving round tie with kitchen string. Peel the garlic cloves and cut into 3 pieces lengthwise. Wash rosemary.
4. Add garlic garlic and rosemary all over the outer surface of the leg of lamb. To do this, make a deep incision with a knife and put inside a piece of garlic and a sprig of rosemary in the background well. Salpimentar generously surface with sea salt and mixing 5 peppers.
5. Peel the potatoes, rinsed and cut into thick slices of 5 mm thickness. Peel onions and cut them into thick equal slices.

6. Grease bottom of the baking tray with olive oil. Place the potato slices on the tray and spread the onion on top.
7. Place the lamb with garlic and rosemary in the center and sprinkle with olive oil.
8. Bake at half height for 15 minutes per 1,1 lb of meat so that little done and 20 to 25 minutes per 1,1 lb to the point that it is either done.
9. A half of cooking, add the potato half glass of water or a little more, as needed.
10. If the surface is browning too quickly, cover with baking paper. Optionally, 15 minutes before end of cooking, sprinkle top with melted butter and finish uncovered.

Nutrition:

Calories: 365

Fat: 21g

Carbs: 11g

Protein: 15g

Roasted Lamb with Honey

Preparation Time: 5 minutes
Cooking Time: 30 minutes
Servings: 4
Ingredients:

- 1,32 lb lamb
- 2 tablespoons mustard tarragon
- 2 tablespoons rosemary honey
- 2 tablespoons soy
- 1 teaspoon rosemary, chopped
- 2 cloves garlic , minced
- C / N Extra virgin olive
- 0,88 lb potatoes , peeled and chopped
- Salt and black pepper

Directions:

1. Put the meat to macerate the night before with mustard, honey, soy, chopped rosemary, garlic, 1 chorretón oil, salt and pepper.
2. Cook the potatoes and Reserve.
3. Place meat in a preheated Air fryer at 392 ° F for 20 '. Remove and add the potatoes.
4. Return to Air fryer and lower the temperature to 338 ° F
5. When the meat is cooked remove and serve with potatoes.

Nutrition:
Calories: 243
Fat: 22g
Carbs: 13g
Protein: 20g

Roasted Lamb with Thyme And Garlic

Preparation Time: 5 minutes
Cooking Time: 30 minutes
Servings: 4
Ingredients:

- 3 pieces of lamb
- 3 cloves of garlic
- olive oil spray
- thyme
- salt pepper

Directions:

1. Season the meat on both sides.
2. Pour a little olive oil spray.
3. Spread crushed garlic on each piece.
4. Preheat airfrer.
5. Put the meat into fryer and add thyme.
6. Wait till meat is fully cooked.
7. Serve.

Nutrition:
Calories: 343
Fat: 7g
Carbs: 6g
Protein: 34g

Chapter 12. Homemade Staples

Cucumber Bites

Preparation Time: 10 minutes
Cooking Time: 0 minutes
Servings: 12
Ingredients:

- 1 English cucumber, sliced into 32 rounds
- 10 ounces hummus
- 16 cherry tomatoes, halved
- 1 tablespoon parsley, chopped
- 1 ounce feta cheese, crumbled

Directions:

1. Spread the hummus on each cucumber round, divide the tomato halves on each, sprinkle the cheese and parsley on to and serve as an appetizer.

Nutrition:
Calories 162;
Fat 3.4 g;
Fiber 2 g;
Carbs 6.4 g;
Protein 2.4 g

Stuffed Avocado

Preparation Time: 10 minutes
Cooking Time: 0 minute
Servings: 2
Ingredients:

- 1 avocado, halved and pitted
- 10 ounces canned tuna, drained
- 2 tablespoons sun-dried tomatoes, chopped
- 1 and ½ tablespoon basil pesto
- 2 tablespoons black olives, pitted and chopped
- Salt and black pepper to the taste
- 2 teaspoons pine nuts, toasted and chopped
- 1 tablespoon basil, chopped

Directions:

1. In a bowl, combine the tuna with the sun-dried tomatoes and the rest of the ingredients except the avocado and stir.
2. Stuff the avocado halves with the tuna mix and serve as an appetizer.

Nutrition:
Calories 233;
Fat 9 g;
Fiber 3.5 g;
Carbs 11.4 g;
Protein 5.6 g

Hummus with Ground Lamb

Preparation Time: 10 minutes
Cooking Time: 15 minute
Servings: 8
Ingredients:

- 10 ounces hummus
- 12 ounces lamb meat, ground
- ½ cup pomegranate seeds
- ¼ cup parsley, chopped
- 1 tablespoon olive oil
- Pita chips for serving

Directions:

1. Heat up a pan with the oil over medium-high heat, add the meat, and brown for 15 minutes stirring often.
2. Spread the hummus on a platter, spread the ground lamb all over, also spread the pomegranate seeds and the parsley and serve with pita chips as a snack.

Nutrition:
Calories 133;
Fat 9.7 g;
Fiber 1.7 g;
Carbs 6.4 g;
Protein 5

Wrapped Plums

Preparation Time: 5 minutes
Cooking Time: 0 minutes
Servings: 8
Ingredients:

- 2 ounces prosciutto, cut into 16 pieces
- 4 plums, quartered
- 1 tablespoon chives, chopped
- A pinch of red pepper flakes, crushed

Directions:

1. Wrap each plum quarter in a prosciutto slice, arrange them all on a platter, sprinkle the chives and pepper flakes all over and serve.

Nutrition:
Calories 30;
Fat 1 g;
Fiber 0 g;
Carbs 4 g;
Protein 2 g

Chapter 13. Poultry

Chicken Stroganoff

Preparation Time: 10 minutes
Cooking Time: 20 minutes
Servings: 4
Ingredients:

- 1 cup cremini mushrooms, sliced
- 1 onion, sliced
- 1 tablespoon olive oil
- ½ teaspoon thyme
- 1 teaspoon salt
- 1 cup Plain yogurt
- 10 oz. chicken fillet, chopped

Directions:

1. Heat up olive oil in the saucepan.
2. Add mushrooms and onion.
3. Sprinkle the vegetables with thyme and salt. Mix up well and cook them for 5 minutes.
4. After this, add chopped chicken fillet and mix up well.
5. Cook the ingredients for 5 minutes more.
6. Then add plain yogurt, mix up well, and close the lid.
7. Cook chicken stroganoff for 10 minutes over the low heat.

Nutrition:
Calories 224,
Fat 9.2 g,
Fiber 0.8 g,
Carbs 7.4 g,
Protein 24.2 g

Pancakes

Preparation Time: 5 minutes
Cooking Time: 6 minutes
Servings: 2
Ingredients

- ¼ cup almond flour
- 1 ½ tbsp. unsalted butter
- 2 oz cream cheese, softened
- 2 eggs

Directions:

1. Take a bowl, crack eggs in it, whisk well until fluffy, and then whisk in flour and cream cheese until well combined.
2. Take a skillet pan, place it over medium heat, add butter and when it melts, drop pancake batter in four sections, spread it evenly, and cook for 2 minutes per side until brown.
3. Serve.

Nutrition:
166.8 Calories;
15 g Fats;
5.8 g Protein;
1.8 g Net Carb;
0.8 g Fiber;

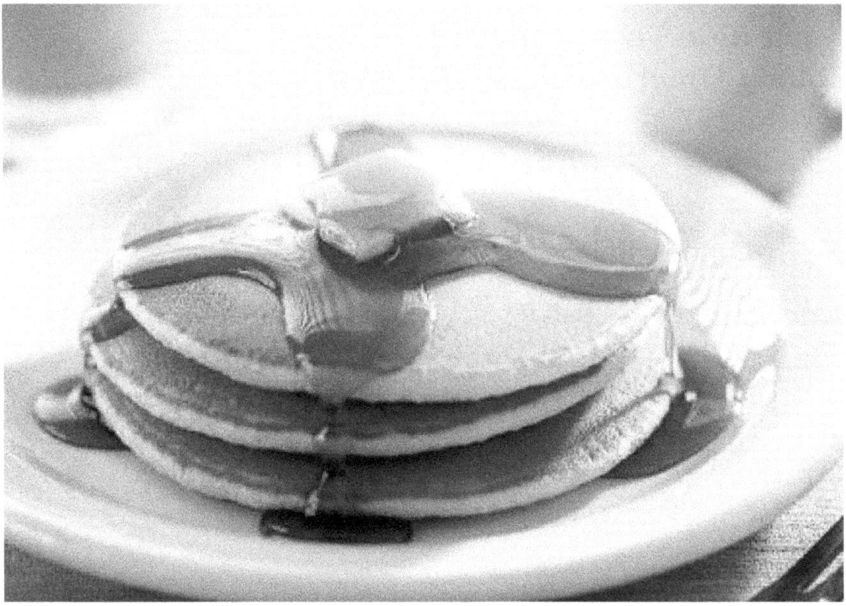

Cheese Roll-Ups

Preparation Time: 5 minutes
Cooking Time: 0 minutes;
Servings: 2
Ingredients

- 2 oz mozzarella cheese, sliced, full-fat
- 1-ounce butter, unsalted

Directions:

1. Cut cheese into slices and then cut butter into thin slices.
2. Top each cheese slice with a slice of butter, roll it and then serve.

Nutrition:
166 Calories;
15 g Fats;
6.5 g Protein;
2 g Net Carb;
0 g Fiber;

Scrambled Eggs with Spinach and Cheese

Preparation Time: 5 minutes
Cooking Time: 5 minutes;
Servings: 2
Ingredients

- 2 oz spinach
- 2 eggs
- 1 tbsp. coconut oil
- 2 tbsp. grated mozzarella cheese, full-fat
- Seasoning:
- ¼ tsp salt
- 1/8 tsp ground black pepper
- 1/8 tsp red pepper flakes

Directions:

1. Take a medium bowl, crack eggs in it, add salt and black pepper and whisk until combined.
2. Take a medium skillet pan, place it over medium heat, add oil and when hot, add spinach and cook for 1 minute until leaves wilt.
3. Pour eggs over spinach, stir and cook for 1 minute until just set.
4. Stir in cheese, then remove the pan from heat and sprinkle red pepper flakes on top.
5. Serve.

Nutrition:
171 Calories;
14 g Fats;
9.2 g Protein;
1.1 g Net Carb;
1.7 g Fiber;

Chapter 14. Fast and Cheap

Norwegian Niçoise Salad: Smoked Salmon, Cucumber, Egg, And Asparagus

Preparation Time: 20 minutes
Cooking Time: 5 minutes
Servings: 4
Ingredients:

- For the vinaigrette
- 3 tablespoons walnut oil
- 2 tablespoons champagne vinegar
- 1 tablespoon chopped fresh dill
- ½ teaspoon kosher salt
- ¼ teaspoon ground mustard
- Freshly ground black pepper

For the salad:

- Handful green beans, trimmed
- 1 (3- to 4-ounce) package spring greens
- 12 spears pickled asparagus
- 4 large soft-boiled eggs, halved
- 8 ounces smoked salmon, thinly sliced
- 1 cucumber, thinly sliced
- 1 lemon, quartered

Directions:

1. To make the dressing
2. In a small bowl, whisk the oil, vinegar, dill, salt, ground mustard, and a few grinds of pepper until emulsified. Set aside.
3. To make the salad
4. Start by blanching the green beans: Bring a pot of salted water to a boil. Drop in the beans. Cook or 1 to 2 minutes until they turn bright green, then immediately drain and rinse under cold water. Set aside.
5. Divide the spring greens among 4 plates. Toss each serving with dressing to taste. Arrange 3 asparagus spears, 1 egg, 2 ounces of salmon, one-fourth of the cucumber slices, and a lemon wedge on each plate. Serve immediately.

Nutrition:

Calories: 257;
Total fat: 18g;
Total carbs: 6g;
Cholesterol: 199mg;
Fiber: 2g;
Protein: 19g;
Sodium: 603mg

Loaded Caesar Salad With Crunchy Chickpeas

Preparation Time: 5 minutes
Cooking Time: 20 minutes
Servings: 6
Ingredients:
For the chickpeas:

- 2 (15-ounce) cans chickpeas, drained and rinsed
- 2 tablespoons extra-virgin olive oil
- 1 teaspoon kosher salt
- 1 teaspoon garlic powder
- 1 teaspoon onion powder
- 1 teaspoon dried oregano

For the dressing:

- ½ cup mayonnaise
- 2 tablespoons grated Parmesan cheese
- 2 tablespoons freshly squeezed lemon juice
- 1 clove garlic, peeled and smashed
- 1 teaspoon Dijon mustard
- ½ tablespoon Worcestershire sauce
- ½ tablespoon anchovy paste

For the salad:

- 3 heads romaine lettuce, cut into bite-size pieces

Directions:

To make the chickpeas:

1. Preheat the oven to 450°F. Line a baking sheet with parchment paper.
2. In a medium bowl, toss together the chickpeas, oil, salt, garlic powder, onion powder, and oregano. Scatter the coated chickpeas on the prepared baking sheet.
3. Roast for about 20 minutes, tossing occasionally, until the chickpeas are golden and have a bit of crunch.

To make the dressing:

1. In a small bowl, whisk the mayonnaise, Parmesan, lemon juice, garlic, mustard, Worcestershire sauce, and anchovy paste until combined.

To make the salad:

2. In a large bowl, combine the lettuce and dressing. Toss to coat. Top with the roasted chickpeas and serve.

Nutrition:

Calories: 367;
Total fat: 22g;
Total carbs: 35g;
Cholesterol: 9mg;
Fiber: 13g;
Protein: 12g;
Sodium: 407mg

Coleslaw Worth A Second Helping

Preparation Time: 20 minutes
Cooking Time: 10 minutes
Servings: 6
Ingredients:

- 5 cups shredded cabbage
- 2 carrots, shredded
- 1/3 cup chopped fresh flat-leaf parsley
- ½ cup mayonnaise
- ½ cup sour cream
- 3 tablespoons apple cider vinegar
- 1 teaspoon kosher salt
- ½ teaspoon celery seed

Directions:

1. In a large bowl, combine the cabbage, carrots, and parsley.
2. In a small bowl, whisk the mayonnaise, sour cream, vinegar, salt, and celery seed until smooth. Pour the dressing over the vegetables and toss until coated. Transfer to a serving bowl and chill until ready to serve.

Nutrition:
Calories: 192;
Total fat: 18g;
Total carbs: 7g;
Cholesterol: 18mg;
Fiber: 3g;
Protein: 2g;
Sodium: 543mg

Chapter 15. Bread

Crispy Sandwich Chaffle

Preparation Time: 3 min
Cooking Time: 4 min
Servings: 1
Ingredients

- 1 egg
- 1/2 cup cheddar cheese, shredded
- 1 tbsp. coconut flour

Directions:

1. Using a mini waffle maker, preheat according to maker's instructions.
2. Combine egg and cheddar cheese in a mixing bowl. Stir thoroughly
3. Add coconut flour for added texture if so desired
4. Place half batter on waffle maker and spread evenly.
5. Cook for 4 minutes or until as desired
6. Gently remove from waffle maker and set aside for 2 minutes so it cools down and become crispy
7. Repeat for remaining batter
8. Stuff 2 chaffles with desired sandwich

Nutrition:
Calories: 363
Protein: 2
Fat: 40
Carbohydrates: 1

Basic Chaffle

Preparation Time: 3 min
Cooking Time: 4 min
Servings: 1
Ingredients

- 1 egg
- 1/2 cup cheddar cheese, shredded
- 1/2 tbsp. Psyllium husk powder
- 1/2 tbsp. chia seeds

Directions:

1. Switch on the waffle maker according to manufacturer's instructions
2. Crack egg and combine with cheddar cheese in a small bowl
3. Place half batter on waffle maker and spread evenly.
4. Sprinkle Chia on top, cover and cook for 4 minutes or until as desired
5. Gently remove from waffle maker and set aside for 2 minutes so it cools down and become crispy
6. Repeat for remaining batter
7. Serve with desired toppings

Nutrition:
Calories: 363
Protein: 2
Fat: 40
Carbohydrates: 1

Sandwich Chaffle

Preparation Time: 3 min
Cooking Time: 4 min
Servings: 1
Ingredients

- 1 egg
- 1/2 cup cheddar cheese, shredded
- 1 tbsp. almond flour (optional)

Directions:

1. Using a mini waffle maker, preheat according to maker's instructions.
2. Combine egg and cheddar cheese in a mixing bowl. Stir thoroughly
3. Add Almond flour for added texture if so desired; mix well
4. Place half batter on waffle maker and spread evenly.
5. Cook for 4 minutes or until as desired
6. Gently remove from waffle maker and set aside for 2 minutes so it cools down and become crispy
7. Repeat for remaining batter
8. Stuff 2 chaffles with desired garnishing to make a sandwich

Nutrition:
170 calories
2g net carbs
14g fat
10g protein

Flaky Delight Chaffle

Preparation Time: 3 min
Cooking Time: 4 min
Servings: 1
Ingredients

- 1 egg
- 1/2 cup cheddar cheese, shredded
- 1/2 cup coconut flakes

Directions:

1. Switch on the waffle maker according to manufacturer's instructions
2. Crack egg and combine with cheddar cheese in a small bowl
3. Place half batter on waffle maker and spread evenly.
4. Sprinkle coconut flakes and Cook for 4 minutes or until as desired
5. Gently remove from waffle maker and set aside for 2 minutes so it cools down and become crispy
6. Repeat for remaining batter
7. Serve with desired toppings

Nutrition:
291 calories
1g net carbs
23g fat
20g protein

Conclusion

Thank you for making it to the end. The Lean and Green Diet can be effectively used for rapid weight loss compared to other plans simply because of the offer made by lean and green meals and its few calories.

This diet depends on strongly confining calories to advance weight reduction. Most "fuelings" drift around 100–110 calories each, which means you could take in about 1,000 calories for every day on this diet.

London concurs that there's a unique way to deal with enduring weight reduction: "'Eating dinners and tidbits that join heaps of produce, 100% entire grains, nuts, seeds, vegetables, and heartbeats, low-Fat: dairy items, eggs, poultry, fish, and lean hamburger in addition to certain extravagances is the most ideal approach to get more fit economically for the long stretch."

You should avoid refined grain, sugar-improved beverages, singed food, and alcohol on the Lean and Green Diet when doing it. During the advancement and upkeep organizes, some carb-containing nourishments are incorporated back in, for instance, low Fat: dairy and new natural products.

The coaching component can be compared to Jenny Craig and Weight Watchers, which urge users to register for meet-ups to get the necessary support. Due to the highly processed nature of the majority of foods available on the Lean and Green Diet, it could pose a threat or challenge compared to the variety of whole, fresh foods you can consume on more self-sustainable plans such as Atkins.

This revolutionary diet enables weight loss through one-on-one coaching, low-carb homemade meals, and low-calorie prepackaged diets. Although the initial 5&1 Plan is quite limiting, the 3&3 maintenance phase enables fewer processed snacks and a wider variety of food, making it easier to lose weight and adhere to the program for sustenance in the long term.

Nevertheless extended calorie restriction may lead to nutrient deficiencies and other risky health concerns.

Although the program promotes Fat: loss and short-term weight loss, further research is required to evaluate the level of lifestyle changes it needs for long-term success.

The bottom line:

The "Lean and Green" weight loss plan promotes weight loss via low-calorie prepackaged meals; quiet carb homemade food, and personalized coaching.

The Lean and Green diet advances weight reduction using low-calorie prepackaged foods, low carb natively constructed suppers, and customized instruction.

However the diet is repetitive and doesn't accommodate all nutritional wishes. What's extra, extended calorie limit may also result in nutrient deficiencies and different potential health issues.

Simultaneously, as this system promotes quick-time period weight and Fat's loss, similarly research is wanted to assess whether it encourages the everlasting way of life adjustments needed for long-time period achievement.

I hope you have learned something!

Lightning Source UK Ltd.
Milton Keynes UK
UKHW020633190421
382237UK00001B/57

9 781802 527629